EPI DIET COOKBOOK

Conquer Chronic Pancreatitis, Inflammation and Pain, Embrace Flavor: Recipes, Meal Plans, and Lifestyle Strategies for New & Experienced Exocrine Pancreatic Insufficiency Patients.

Harper Bloom

TABLE OF CONTENTS

Reclaiming the Kitchen with EPI

Imagine the joy of whipping up a delicious meal in your own kitchen. The sizzle of lean protein in a pan, the vibrant colors of fresh vegetables being chopped, the anticipation of a satisfying and healthy dish. This used to be a daily ritual for David, but after his EPI diagnosis, the kitchen became a battleground. Fatty foods triggered discomfort, and navigating dietary restrictions felt overwhelming.

Across the country, a similar story unfolded for Maya. Diagnosed with EPI in her late fifties, she found traditional recipes packed with hidden triggers. The thought of cooking became a source of stress, replacing the pleasure she once derived from creating meals for herself and loved ones.

David and Maya's experiences are all too common. Exocrine Pancreatitis Insufficiency (EPI) disrupts digestion, leaving many struggling with pain and nutrient deficiencies. The fear of triggering these symptoms can turn mealtimes into a challenge, robbing individuals of the joy of cooking and sharing food.

This cookbook is for David, Maya, and everyone else who wants to reclaim the kitchen with EPI. Here, you'll find delicious and approachable recipes specifically designed for the EPI diet. We'll focus on low-fat, low-fiber ingredients bursting with flavor and essential nutrients. We'll provide clear instructions and substitution suggestions, empowering you to create satisfying meals with confidence.

Whether you're newly diagnosed or a seasoned EPI warrior, this book equips you to navigate the world of food with newfound freedom. We'll explore the science behind EPI, offer meal planning strategies, and celebrate the possibilities that come with a well-managed condition.

Let's embark on this culinary journey together, transforming your kitchen from a source of anxiety into a space for creativity, delicious exploration, and the joy of nourishing yourself and those you love.

Chapter One

Understanding Exocrine Pancreatic Insufficiency (EPI)

What is Exocrine Pancreatic Insufficiency (EPI)?

Imagine your pancreas as a tiny kitchen in your belly. Its job is to whip up special digestive juices (enzymes) that break down your food – like proteins, fats, and carbs – into smaller pieces. These tiny pieces are then easily absorbed by your intestines, delivering essential nutrients to your body.

Exocrine Pancreatic Insufficiency (EPI) happens when your pancreas isn't producing enough of these digestive juices. Without them, your food doesn't get broken down properly, leading to a variety of unpleasant symptoms and making it hard for your body to absorb the good stuff it needs.

Causes and Risk Factors of EPI

Several things can put your pancreas under strain and lead to EPI. Some common culprits include:

- **Chronic Pancreatitis:** This is like a long-term tummy ache in your pancreas, causing damage that affects enzyme production.

- **Cystic Fibrosis:** This genetic condition affects various organs, including the pancreas, leading to problems with enzyme production.

- **Surgery:** Sometimes, surgeries involving the pancreas or stomach can affect enzyme production.

- **Rare Cases:** In some rare situations, the way your pancreas is built can affect how well it makes enzymes.

Here are some things that can increase your chances of developing EPI:

- **Smoking:** Cigarettes are bad news for your pancreas, just like they are for your lungs.

- **Heavy Drinking:** Overdoing alcohol can damage your pancreas and contribute to EPI.

- **Autoimmune Diseases:** In some cases, your body's defense system can mistakenly attack the pancreas, leading to EPI.

Symptoms of EPI

The symptoms of EPI can vary from person to person, and they might creep up slowly over time. Some of the most common ones include:

- **Oily, smelly stools:** Undigested fats can make your bowel movements oily and unpleasant.

- **Going to the bathroom more often:** Since your body can't absorb everything from your food, you might experience more frequent bowel movements.

- **Belly pain and cramps:** Undigested food moving through your intestines too quickly can cause discomfort and cramping.

- **Feeling bloated and gassy:** Difficulty digesting certain foods, like carbohydrates, can lead to bloating and gas.

- **Losing weight without trying:** Because your body struggles to absorb nutrients from food, you might experience unintended weight loss.

- **Feeling tired and weak:** The lack of proper nutrient absorption can make you feel fatigued and lacking in energy.

If you're experiencing any of these symptoms for a while, it's important to talk to your doctor. They can help figure out what's going on and discuss the best treatment options.

Diagnosis of EPI

Diagnosing EPI often involves a combination of detective work by your doctor. They'll likely ask about your medical history and symptoms, do a physical exam, and might order some tests like:

- **Stool tests:** These check your poop for signs of excess fat, which can be a clue for EPI.

- **Blood tests:** While not always definitive, certain blood tests can measure levels of pancreatic enzymes.

- **Imaging tests:** X-rays, CT scans, or MRIs can give your doctor a clearer picture of your pancreas and see if anything looks off.

- **Secretin stimulation test:** This test helps see how well your pancreas responds to a special hormone that triggers enzyme production.

Getting an early diagnosis and managing EPI properly is key to feeling better and preventing complications. This cookbook will be your partner on this journey, providing delicious recipes and information to help you navigate an EPI diet with confidence!

Chapter Two

Living Well with EPI

Now that you understand EPI, let's delve into how to live a full and enjoyable life while managing this condition. This chapter explores the connections between EPI, inflammation, and pain, and equips you with essential knowledge about enzymes, meal planning, and portion control.

The Link Between EPI, Chronic Pancreatitis, Inflammation, and Pain

Chronic Pancreatitis: Sometimes referred to as long-term inflammation of the pancreas, chronic pancreatitis can damage the cells responsible for producing digestive enzymes. This damage can lead to EPI.

Inflammation: When your pancreas is inflamed, it can trigger the release of substances that irritate nearby tissues, causing pain.

In EPI, undigested food passing through the intestines can also contribute to inflammation and discomfort.

Pain: Abdominal pain is a frequent symptom of EPI, often linked to inflammation and the difficulty your digestive system has processing food.

The Takeaway: While chronic pancreatitis can lead to EPI, not everyone with EPI will have experienced pancreatitis. However, managing inflammation through diet and medication can significantly improve your comfort and overall well-being.

Understanding Enzymes and Enzyme Replacement Therapy (ERT)

Enzymes: As mentioned earlier, your pancreas produces enzymes that break down proteins, fats, and carbohydrates in your food.

Enzyme Replacement Therapy (ERT): Since your body struggles to produce enough enzymes with EPI, ERT is a crucial part of managing the condition.

These medications, taken with meals and snacks, replace the missing enzymes and aid digestion.

Taking ERT Effectively:

- Follow your doctor's instructions regarding dosage and timing.

- Take ERT with every meal and snack containing protein or fat.

- ERT capsules should be swallowed whole, not crushed or chewed.

Important Note: ERT medications work by aiding digestion, but they don't cure EPI.

Importance of Nutrition for People with EPI

A healthy diet is essential for everyone, but it becomes even more important when managing EPI. Proper nutrition helps:

- **Reduce Symptoms:** By choosing foods your body can easily digest, you can minimize discomfort and inflammation.

- **Absorb Nutrients:** A well-balanced EPI diet ensures you get the vitamins and minerals your body needs to function optimally.

- **Maintain Weight:** EPI can lead to weight loss. Focusing on nutrient-rich foods helps you maintain a healthy weight.

Meal Planning and Portion Control for EPI

Planning your meals and controlling portions are key strategies for managing EPI effectively. Here are some tips:

- **Plan Your Meals:** Having a plan reduces the stress of figuring out what to eat on the fly, potentially leading to unhealthy choices.

- **Focus on Low-Fat Options:** Choose lean protein sources like grilled chicken, fish, or beans. Limit fried foods and fatty cuts of meat.

- **Mind Your Fiber:** While fiber is essential for overall health, too much can interfere with enzyme function.

Opt for lower-fiber vegetables and fruits, or cook them thoroughly to soften the fiber content.

- **Portion Control is Key:** Eating smaller, more frequent meals can be easier for your digestive system to handle compared to large, heavy meals.

- **Don't Forget Hydration:** Staying hydrated is crucial for digestion and overall health. Aim for water throughout the day.

By incorporating these strategies and the delicious recipes in this book, you can create a sustainable and enjoyable approach to managing EPI.

Chapter Three

Navigating the EPI Diet: Making Delicious Choices for a Healthy You

The EPI diet prioritizes foods that are easily digested and nutrient-rich, helping you manage symptoms and feel your best. Here's a breakdown of the core principles and what to include (and avoid) on your EPI plate.

General Principles:

- **Eat Smaller Meals More Often:** Aim for 5-6 smaller meals and snacks throughout the day. This reduces stress on your digestive system and allows for better nutrient absorption.

- **Embrace Low-Fat Options:** Limit fried foods, processed meats, and fatty cuts of meat. Choose lean protein sources like grilled chicken, fish, or beans.

- **Fiber in Moderation:** While fiber is important for overall health, too much can interfere with enzyme function in EPI. Opt for lower-fiber fruits and vegetables or cook them thoroughly to soften the fiber content.

- **Portion Control is Key:** Focus on smaller portions to avoid overwhelming your digestive system.

- **Stay Hydrated:** Drinking plenty of water throughout the day is crucial for digestion and overall health.

- **Don't Forget Supplements:** Talk to your doctor about vitamin and mineral supplements to ensure you're getting the nutrients your body needs.

- **Limit Alcohol and Smoking:** Excessive alcohol consumption can worsen EPI symptoms. Smoking is also a risk factor for chronic pancreatitis, a leading cause of EPI.

- **Enzyme Replacement Therapy:** Remember to take your pancreatic enzyme replacement therapy with every meal and snack containing protein or fat, as prescribed by your doctor.

- **Listen to Your Body:** Sometimes, you may need to rest and prioritize digestion. Don't be afraid to adjust your meal schedule or portion sizes based on how you're feeling.

Foods to Choose On (Low-Fat, Low-Fiber, Nutrient-Rich):

- **Lean Protein Powerhouses:** Chicken, turkey, fish, eggs, and lentils provide essential protein while being low in unhealthy fats.

- **Healthy Fat Choices:** Incorporate heart-healthy unsaturated fats from nuts, seeds, olive oil, avocado, and fatty fish like salmon.

- **Colorful Fruits and Veggies:** Enjoy a variety of fresh fruits and vegetables, opting for lower-fiber options or cooking them thoroughly when necessary.

- **Simple Salad Dressings:** Opt for light dressings like vinegar or fresh lemon juice instead of creamy options.

- **Veggie Sides:** Choose steamed or roasted vegetables over french fries or potato chips.

- **Light Appetizers:** Clear soups, steamed clams, or shrimp cocktail are gentle on your digestive system.

- **Refreshing Desserts:** Sorbet or fresh fruit makes a delightful and low-fat dessert option.

Foods to Limit (High-Fat, High-Fiber):

- **Processed Foods:** Limit processed foods like pre-packaged snacks, fatty cuts of meat, and fried foods.

- **High-Fiber Fruits and Vegetables:** While fruits and vegetables are essential, some can be high in fiber. Choose options like applesauce, peeled potatoes, or cooked greens.

- **Heavy Meals:** Large meals can overwhelm your digestive system. Opt for smaller, more frequent meals throughout the day.

- **Alcohol:** It's best to avoid alcohol or consume it in strict moderation, as it can worsen EPI symptoms.

Sample EPI Meal Plans:

Sample 1-Day Meal Plan:

- **Breakfast:** Scrambled eggs with chopped peppers and low-fat cheese, whole-wheat toast

- **Lunch:** Tuna salad sandwich on whole-wheat bread with lettuce and tomato, side salad with vinaigrette dressing

- **Dinner:** Baked salmon with roasted vegetables, brown rice

- **Snacks:** Low-fat yogurt with berries, handful of almonds

Sample 3-Day Meal Plan:

- **Day 1:** Breakfast - Oatmeal with berries and walnuts, Lunch - Chicken breast salad with mixed greens and light vinaigrette, Dinner - Turkey burgers on sweet potato buns with roasted vegetables

- **Day 2:** Breakfast - Smoothie made with low-fiber fruits, protein powder, and almond milk, Lunch -

Lentil soup with whole-wheat bread, Dinner - Baked cod with steamed broccoli and quinoa

- **Day 3:** Breakfast - Eggs with whole-wheat toast and avocado slices, Lunch - Grilled chicken Caesar salad with light dressing (hold the croutons), Dinner - Shrimp stir-fry with brown rice and low-fiber vegetables

Sample 1-Week Meal Plan:

This provides a general structure, allowing you to swap in your favorite EPI-friendly choices throughout the week.

- **Breakfast Ideas:** Scrambled eggs, oatmeal, whole-wheat pancakes with fruit, yogurt parfait with granola

- **Lunch Ideas:** Grilled chicken or fish sandwiches on whole-wheat bread, Soup and salad combinations, lentil or bean salads, tuna or chicken salad wraps

- **Dinner Ideas:** Baked chicken or fish with roasted vegetables, turkey burgers on sweet potato buns, vegetarian chili with cornbread, lentil soup with whole-wheat bread, stir-fries with lean protein and low-fiber vegetables

- **Snack Ideas:** Fresh fruits with nut butter, low-fat yogurt with berries, vegetable sticks with hummus, hard-boiled eggs, handful of almonds or walnuts

- **Remember:** These are just samples. Feel free to personalize your meals based on your preferences and what works best for your body. This cookbook offers a variety of recipes specifically designed for the EPI diet, providing you with the inspiration and tools to create delicious and satisfying meals throughout the week.

Chapter Four

EPI-Friendly Breakfast Delights:

Start your day with delicious and nourishing breakfasts that are gentle on your digestive system. These recipes prioritize lean protein, low-fiber options, and heart-healthy fats, keeping you energized and comfortable throughout the morning.

1. Scrambled Eggs with Smoked Salmon and Asparagus

This protein-packed breakfast is bursting with flavor. Smoked salmon adds a touch of luxury, while asparagus provides a welcome pop of green.

Ingredients:

- 2 large eggs
- 1 tablespoon unsweetened almond milk
- Salt and pepper to taste

- 1 tablespoon olive oil

- 2 ounces smoked salmon, thinly sliced

- 4 asparagus spears, trimmed and chopped

Instructions:

1. In a bowl, whisk together eggs, almond milk, salt, and pepper.

2. Heat olive oil in a non-stick pan over medium heat. Add the asparagus and cook for 2-3 minutes, until slightly tender-crisp.

3. Push the asparagus to the side of the pan. Pour in the egg mixture and scramble gently until cooked through.

4. Fold in the smoked salmon and heat for another minute.

5. Serve immediately.

Nutritional Information (per serving):

- Calories: 280

- Protein: 18g

- Fat: 15g

- Carbs: 5g

2. Berry Smoothie with Protein Powder

This quick and refreshing smoothie is a great way to start your day with a blend of protein, vitamins, and healthy fats.

Ingredients:

- 1 cup frozen mixed berries

- 1/2 cup unsweetened almond milk

- 1 scoop vanilla protein powder

- 1/4 cup plain, low-fat Greek yogurt

- 1/4 cup water (optional, adjust for desired consistency)

Instructions:

1. Combine all ingredients in a blender and blend until smooth and creamy.

2. Add a little water if the mixture is too thick.

3. Pour into a glass and enjoy!

Nutritional Information (per serving):

- Calories: 250

- Protein: 20g

- Fat: 5g

- Carbs: 20g

3. Whole-Wheat Pancakes with Ricotta and Berries

These fluffy pancakes are a delicious and satisfying way to fuel your morning. Whole-wheat flour adds fiber, while ricotta cheese provides a creamy protein boost.

Ingredients:

- 1 cup whole-wheat flour

- 1 teaspoon baking powder

- 1/4 teaspoon salt

- 1 cup unsweetened almond milk

- 1 egg

- 1 tablespoon olive oil

- 1/4 cup ricotta cheese

- 1/2 cup fresh berries

Instructions:

1. In a medium bowl, whisk together flour, baking powder, and salt.

2. In a separate bowl, whisk together almond milk, egg, and olive oil.

3. Fold the wet ingredients into the dry ingredients until just combined. Do not overmix.

4. Heat a lightly greased non-stick pan over medium heat. Pour batter into 1/4 cup portions to make pancakes.

5. Cook for 2-3 minutes per side, or until golden brown and cooked through.

6. Top with ricotta cheese and fresh berries.

Nutritional Information (per serving with ricotta and berries):

- Calories: 350

- Protein: 15g

- Fat: 12g

- Carbs: 40g

4. Baked Egg Cups with Spinach and Feta

These individual egg cups are a healthy and portable breakfast option. Packed with protein and vegetables, they'll keep you satisfied until lunchtime.

Ingredients:

- 4 large eggs

- 1/2 cup chopped spinach

- 1/4 cup crumbled feta cheese

- 1/4 cup chopped cherry tomatoes

- Salt and pepper to taste

Instructions:

1. Preheat oven to 375°F (190°C). Grease a muffin tin or use silicone muffin cups.

2. Divide spinach, feta cheese, and cherry tomatoes evenly among the muffin cups.

3. Crack an egg into each muffin cup. Season with salt and pepper.

4. Bake for 15-20 minutes, or until egg whites are set and yolks are cooked to your preference.

5. Let cool slightly before serving.

Nutritional Information (per serving):

- Calories: 220

- Protein: 12g

- Fat: 10g

- Carbs: 5g

5. Chia Seed Pudding with Berries

This overnight oats-inspired breakfast is packed with fiber and protein, making it a slow-digesting and satisfying option.

Ingredients:

- 1/3 cup chia seeds

- 1 cup unsweetened almond milk

- 1/4 teaspoon vanilla extract

- 1/4 cup fresh or frozen berries

- Optional toppings: Sliced almonds, chopped nuts, shredded coconut

Instructions:

1. In a bowl or jar, whisk together chia seeds, almond milk, and vanilla extract.

2. Cover and refrigerate overnight or for at least 8 hours.

3. In the morning, stir in fresh or frozen berries.

4. Top with your favorite toppings like sliced almonds, chopped nuts, or shredded coconut (optional).

Nutritional Information (per serving):

- Calories: 280

- Protein: 5g

- Fat: 12g

- Carbs: 25g

6. Turkey Sausage Frittata with Roasted Peppers

This savory frittata is a protein-rich and flavorful breakfast option. Pre-roasted peppers add a touch of sweetness and vibrant color.

Ingredients:

- 4 eggs

- 1/4 cup unsweetened almond milk

- 1/4 cup chopped cooked turkey sausage

- 1/2 cup chopped roasted red peppers (from a jar or roasted fresh)

- 1/4 cup crumbled feta cheese

- Salt and pepper to taste

- 1 tablespoon olive oil

Instructions:

1. Preheat oven to 375°F (190°C). Grease a small oven-safe skillet or pie dish.

2. In a bowl, whisk together eggs and almond milk. Season with salt and pepper.

3. Heat olive oil in the skillet over medium heat. Add the cooked turkey sausage and cook for 1-2 minutes, until slightly browned.

4. Pour in the egg mixture and sprinkle with roasted peppers and feta cheese.

5. Bake for 20-25 minutes, or until the eggs are set and the center is cooked through.

6. Let cool slightly before serving.

Nutritional Information (per serving):

- Calories: 300

- Protein: 20g

- Fat: 15g

- Carbs: 5g

7. Greek Yogurt Parfait with Granola and Berries

This layered parfait is a beautiful and delicious way to start your day. Creamy Greek yogurt provides protein, while granola adds a touch of sweetness and crunch.

Ingredients:

- 1/2 cup plain, low-fat Greek yogurt

- 1/4 cup granola (choose a low-fiber option)

- 1/2 cup fresh berries

- 1 tablespoon chopped nuts (optional)

Instructions:

1. In a parfait glass or bowl, layer half of the Greek yogurt, followed by half of the granola and half of the berries.

2. Repeat with another layer of yogurt, granola, and berries.

3. Top with chopped nuts (optional).

Nutritional Information (per serving):

- Calories: 250

- Protein: 15g

- Fat: 7g

- Carbs: 25g

8. Egg Muffins with Ham and Vegetables

This recipe offers another variation on baked egg cups, packed with protein and savory flavor.

Ingredients:

- 4 large eggs

- 1/4 cup chopped cooked ham

- 1/4 cup chopped bell peppers

- 1/4 cup chopped mushrooms

- 1/4 cup shredded mozzarella cheese

- Salt and pepper to taste

Instructions:

1. Preheat oven to 375°F (190°C). Grease a muffin tin or use silicone muffin cups.

2. Divide cooked ham, bell peppers, and mushrooms evenly among the muffin cups.

3. Crack an egg into each muffin cup. Season with salt and pepper.

4. Sprinkle with shredded mozzarella cheese.

5. Bake for 15-20 minutes, or until egg whites are set and yolks are cooked to your preference.

6. Let cool slightly before serving.

Nutritional Information (per serving):

- Calories: 250

- Protein: 15g

- Fat: 12g

- Carbs: 5g

9. Sweet Potato Toast with Avocado and Eggs

This trendy breakfast option gets a makeover for the EPI diet. Sweet potato provides complex carbohydrates and vitamins, while avocado adds healthy fats and creaminess.

Ingredients:

- 1 small sweet potato, sliced into 1/4-inch thick rounds

- 1/2 avocado, mashed

- 2 large eggs

- Salt and pepper to taste

- Optional toppings: Chopped fresh herbs (such as chives, parsley, or cilantro)

Instructions:

1. Preheat oven to 400°F (200°C). Line a baking sheet with parchment paper.

2. Arrange sweet potato slices on the prepared baking sheet. Brush lightly with olive oil (optional).

3. Bake for 20-25 minutes, flipping halfway through, or until tender-crisp.

4. While the sweet potato is baking, cook your eggs according to your preference (fried, scrambled, poached). Season with salt and pepper.

5. Once the sweet potato slices are cooked, spread mashed avocado on each slice.

6. Top with a cooked egg and sprinkle with chopped fresh herbs (optional).

Nutritional Information (per serving):

- Calories: 300

- Protein: 8g

- Fat: 15g

- Carbs: 30g

10. Protein Pancakes with Berries and Nut Butter

This recipe provides a fluffy pancake option with a protein boost. Nut butter adds a touch of healthy fat and extra protein.

Ingredients:

- 1 cup whole-wheat flour

- 1 scoop vanilla protein powder

- 1 teaspoon baking powder

- 1/4 teaspoon salt

- 1 1/4 cups unsweetened almond milk

- 1 tablespoon olive oil

- 1 egg

- 1/2 cup fresh berries

- 2 tablespoons nut butter (such as almond butter or peanut butter)

Instructions:

1. In a medium bowl, whisk together flour, protein powder, baking powder, and salt.

2. In a separate bowl, whisk together almond milk, olive oil, and egg.

3. Fold the wet ingredients into the dry ingredients until just combined. Do not overmix.

4. Heat a lightly greased non-stick pan over medium heat. Pour batter into 1/4 cup portions to make pancakes.

5. Cook for 2-3 minutes per side, or until golden brown and cooked through.

6. Serve pancakes with fresh berries and a dollop of nut butter.

Nutritional Information (per serving with berries and nut butter):

- Calories: 400

- Protein: 25g

- Fat: 15g

- Carbs: 35g

These EPI-friendly breakfast recipes offer a variety of delicious and satisfying options to start your day. Remember to personalize these recipes based on your preferences and what works best for your body. Enjoy!

Chapter Five

EPI-Friendly Lunchbox Delights:

Packing a delicious and nutritious lunch is easy with these EPI-friendly recipes. They focus on portability, ease of preparation, and lean protein sources, keeping you fueled and satisfied throughout the afternoon.

1. Curried Chicken Salad with Grapes and Almonds

This flavorful chicken salad features a light curry dressing and a touch of sweetness from grapes. Almonds add a satisfying crunch.

Ingredients:

- 2 cups cooked, shredded chicken breast
- 1/4 cup mayonnaise (low-fat or Greek yogurt)
- 1 tablespoon curry powder
- 1 tablespoon raisins or dried cranberries (chopped)

- 1/4 cup red grapes, halved

- 1/4 cup sliced almonds

- Salt and pepper to taste

- 2 slices whole-wheat bread

Instructions:

1. In a bowl, combine shredded chicken, mayonnaise, curry powder, raisins, grapes, and almonds.

2. Season with salt and pepper to taste.

3. Divide the chicken salad mixture between two slices of whole-wheat bread.

Nutritional Information (per serving):

- Calories: 400

- Protein: 30g

- Fat: 10g

- Carbs: 30g

2. Turkey and Veggie Wrap with Hummus

This wrap is packed with protein and vegetables, making it a well-balanced and satisfying lunch option. Hummus adds a creamy texture and healthy fats.

Ingredients:

- 4 ounces sliced turkey breast

- 1 large romaine lettuce leaf

- 1/4 cup chopped cucumber

- 1/4 cup shredded carrots

- 1/4 cup hummus

- Salt and pepper to taste

- 1 whole-wheat tortilla

Instructions:

1. Spread hummus evenly on the whole-wheat tortilla.

2. Layer turkey breast, cucumber, and carrots on top of the hummus.

3. Season with salt and pepper to taste.

4. Wrap the tortilla tightly.

Nutritional Information (per serving):

- Calories: 350

- Protein: 25g

- Fat: 10g

- Carbs: 30g

3. Leftover Baked Salmon with Roasted Vegetables

Leftovers make for a perfect EPI-friendly lunch! Baked salmon is a great source of lean protein, and roasted vegetables add essential vitamins and fiber.

Ingredients:

- 2-3 ounces leftover baked salmon

- 1/2 cup leftover roasted vegetables (such as broccoli, carrots, asparagus)

- Side salad with vinaigrette dressing (optional)

- Whole-wheat crackers (optional)

Instructions:

1. Pack leftover baked salmon and roasted vegetables in a container.

2. If desired, include a side salad with a light vinaigrette dressing and some whole-wheat crackers for added crunch.

Nutritional Information (varies depending on leftover recipe):

- This will depend on the specific recipe used for baking the salmon and vegetables. However, a typical serving of baked salmon is around 200 calories with 20g protein and 5g fat. Roasted vegetables typically range from 25-50 calories per cup.

4. Tuna Salad Lettuce Cups with Bell Pepper and Celery

A lighter take on tuna salad, this recipe uses lettuce cups instead of bread and incorporates colorful bell peppers and celery for added flavor and crunch.

Ingredients:

- 1 can (5 oz) water-packed tuna, drained

- 2 tablespoons mayonnaise (low-fat or Greek yogurt)

- 1/4 cup chopped red bell pepper

- 1/4 cup chopped celery

- 1 tablespoon chopped fresh chives

- Salt and pepper to taste

- 4 large romaine lettuce leaves

Instructions:

1. In a bowl, combine tuna, mayonnaise, red bell pepper, celery, and chives.

2. Season with salt and pepper to taste.

3. Fill each romaine lettuce leaf with the tuna salad mixture.

Nutritional Information (per serving):

- Calories: 250

- Protein: 20g

- Fat: 5g

- Carbs: 5g

5. Chicken Kabobs with Tzatziki Sauce

Marinated chicken chunks are skewered with vegetables and grilled to perfection. Tzatziki sauce adds a cool and refreshing touch.

Ingredients:

- 1 pound boneless, skinless chicken breasts, cut into cubes

- 1 tablespoon olive oil

- 1 tablespoon lemon juice

- 1/2 teaspoon dried oregano

- 1/4 teaspoon garlic powder

- 1/4 teaspoon salt

- 1/4 teaspoon black pepper

- 1 red bell pepper, cut into chunks

- 1 green bell pepper, cut into chunks

- 1 red onion, cut into wedges

- 1 container (16 ounces) Greek yogurt, plain nonfat

- 1 small cucumber, seeded and grated

- 1 tablespoon olive oil

- 1 clove garlic, minced

- 1/2 teaspoon dried dill weed

- Pita bread (optional)

Instructions:

1. In a bowl, combine olive oil, lemon juice, oregano, garlic powder, salt, and pepper. Add chicken cubes and marinate for at least 30 minutes.

2. Preheat grill to medium-high heat. Thread chicken cubes, bell peppers, and red onion onto skewers.

3. Grill kabobs for 10-15 minutes per side, or until chicken is cooked through.

4. In a separate bowl, combine Greek yogurt, cucumber, olive oil, garlic, and dill weed.

5. Serve kabobs with tzatziki sauce and pita bread (optional).

Nutritional Information (per serving without pita bread):

- Calories: 400

- Protein: 35g

- Fat: 15g

- Carbs: 15g

6. Lentil Soup with Whole-Wheat Bread

This hearty soup is packed with protein and fiber from lentils. It's a nourishing and satisfying lunch option.

Ingredients:

- 1 tablespoon olive oil

- 1 onion, chopped

- 2 carrots, chopped

- 2 celery stalks, chopped

- 2 cloves garlic, minced

- 1 cup green lentils, rinsed

- 4 cups low-sodium chicken broth

- 1 (14.5 oz) can diced tomatoes, undrained

- 1 teaspoon dried thyme

- 1/2 teaspoon salt

- 1/4 teaspoon black pepper

- 2 slices whole-wheat bread

Instructions:

1. Heat olive oil in a large pot over medium heat. Add onion, carrots, and celery. Cook for 5 minutes, or until softened.

2. Add garlic and cook for an additional minute.

3. Stir in lentils, chicken broth, diced tomatoes, thyme, salt, and pepper. Bring to a boil, then reduce heat and simmer for 30-35 minutes, or until lentils are tender.

4. Serve soup hot with slices of whole-wheat bread.

Nutritional Information (per serving):

- Calories: 350

- Protein: 18g

- Fat: 5g

- Carbs: 50g

7. Leftover Shrimp Scampi over Whole-Wheat Pasta

Leftovers can be transformed into a delicious lunch! Shrimp scampi with a light sauce is perfect served over whole-wheat pasta.

Ingredients:

- 2-3 ounces leftover shrimp scampi with a light sauce

- 1/2 cup cooked whole-wheat pasta

- Side salad with vinaigrette dressing (optional)

Instructions:

1. Pack leftover shrimp scampi and cooked whole-wheat pasta in separate containers.

2. If desired, include a side salad with a light vinaigrette dressing.

Nutritional Information (varies depending on leftover recipe):

- This will depend on the specific recipe used for shrimp scampi. However, a typical serving of shrimp scampi is around 300 calories with 25g protein and 10g fat. A serving of whole-wheat pasta is typically around 200 calories with 8g protein and 40g carbs.

8. Turkey and Avocado Roll-Ups with Whole-Wheat Tortillas

This is a quick and easy lunch option that's perfect for busy days. Turkey, avocado, and lettuce provide a satisfying combination of protein, healthy fats, and fiber.

Ingredients:

- 4 ounces sliced turkey breast

- 1 large romaine lettuce leaf

- 1/2 avocado, mashed

- 1 tablespoon light mayonnaise (optional)

- 1/4 cup shredded carrots

- 1/4 cup chopped cucumber

- 1 whole-wheat tortilla

Instructions:

1. Spread mashed avocado (and mayonnaise, if using) evenly on the whole-wheat tortilla.

2. Layer romaine lettuce leaf, sliced turkey breast, shredded carrots, and chopped cucumber on top of the avocado mixture.

3. Roll the tortilla tightly to enclose the filling.

4. Cut the roll-up in half for easier eating.

Nutritional Information (per serving):

- Calories: 400

- Protein: 30g

- Fat: 15g

- Carbs: 25g

9. Egg Salad with Whole-Wheat Crackers and Grapes

This classic lunch option gets an EPI-friendly makeover. Whole-wheat crackers provide a satisfying crunch, while grapes add a touch of sweetness.

Ingredients:

- 2 hard-boiled eggs, chopped

- 2 tablespoons mayonnaise (low-fat or Greek yogurt)

- 1/4 teaspoon dried mustard powder

- Salt and pepper to taste

- 1/4 cup red grapes

- 1/4 cup whole-wheat crackers

Instructions:

1. In a bowl, combine chopped eggs, mayonnaise, mustard powder, salt, and pepper.

2. Fold in red grapes.

3. Serve egg salad with whole-wheat crackers.

Nutritional Information (per serving):

- Calories: 300

- Protein: 15g

- Fat: 10g

- Carbs: 25g

10. Chicken and Vegetable Power Bowl

This protein-packed bowl is full of flavor and nutrients. Leftover grilled chicken, quinoa, and roasted vegetables come together for a satisfying lunch.

Ingredients:

- 2-3 ounces cooked, shredded chicken breast

- 1/2 cup cooked quinoa

- 1/2 cup roasted vegetables (such as broccoli, carrots, bell peppers)

- 1/4 cup cherry tomatoes, halved

- 1 tablespoon olive oil

- 1 tablespoon lemon juice

- 1/4 teaspoon dried oregano

- Salt and pepper to taste

Instructions:

1. In a bowl, combine cooked chicken, quinoa, roasted vegetables, and cherry tomatoes.

2. In a separate bowl, whisk together olive oil, lemon juice, oregano, salt, and pepper.

3. Drizzle the dressing over the chicken and vegetable mixture.

4. Toss to coat and serve.

Nutritional Information (per serving):

- Calories: 400

- Protein: 30g

- Fat: 10g

- Carbs: 40g

These EPI-friendly lunch recipes offer a variety of delicious and portable options to fuel your afternoons. Remember to personalize these recipes based on your preferences and what works best for your body. Enjoy!

Chapter Six

EPI-Friendly Dinner Delights:

These recipes offer a delicious and satisfying way to end your day while staying mindful of your EPI diet. They explore various protein sources and cooking methods, incorporating lean meats, fish, and vegetables in a low-fiber and easily digestible way.

1. Lemon Herb Baked Cod with Asparagus and Quinoa

This light and flavorful dish features flaky cod baked with a refreshing lemon herb sauce. Asparagus and quinoa add a touch of color and complex carbohydrates.

Ingredients:

- 2 cod fillets (around 6 oz each)

- 1 tablespoon olive oil

- 1 tablespoon lemon juice

- 1/2 teaspoon dried thyme

- 1/4 teaspoon garlic powder

- Salt and pepper to taste

- 1 cup cooked quinoa

- 1 bunch asparagus, trimmed and cut into 1-inch pieces

Instructions:

1. Preheat oven to 400°F (200°C). Lightly grease a baking dish.

2. In a small bowl, whisk together olive oil, lemon juice, thyme, garlic powder, salt, and pepper.

3. Place cod fillets in the prepared baking dish. Pour the lemon herb sauce over the cod.

4. Arrange asparagus spears around the cod.

5. Bake for 15-20 minutes, or until cod is cooked through and flakes easily with a fork.

6. Serve cod with roasted asparagus and cooked quinoa.

Nutritional Information (per serving):

- Calories: 400

- Protein: 30g

- Fat: 10g

- Carbs: 35g

2. Turkey Meatloaf with Roasted Brussels Sprouts

This recipe offers a healthier twist on a classic comfort food. Lean ground turkey forms the base of the meatloaf, while roasted Brussels sprouts add a touch of sweetness and essential vitamins.

Ingredients:

- 1 pound lean ground turkey

- 1/2 cup panko breadcrumbs

- 1/4 cup chopped onion

- 1 egg, beaten

- 1 tablespoon ketchup

- 1 teaspoon Worcestershire sauce

- 1/2 teaspoon dried thyme

- Salt and pepper to taste

- 1 pound Brussels sprouts, trimmed and halved

- 1 tablespoon olive oil

Instructions:

1. Preheat oven to 400°F (200°C). Line a baking sheet with parchment paper.

2. In a large bowl, combine ground turkey, panko breadcrumbs, onion, egg, ketchup, Worcestershire sauce, thyme, salt, and pepper. Mix well to combine.

3. Form the turkey mixture into a loaf shape and place on the prepared baking sheet.

4. Toss Brussels sprouts with olive oil and spread them around the meatloaf.

5. Bake for 40-45 minutes, or until the meatloaf is cooked through and the Brussels sprouts are tender-crisp.

Nutritional Information (per serving):

- Calories: 450

- Protein: 40g

- Fat: 15g

- Carbs: 30g

3. Poached Chicken with Roasted Sweet Potato and Green Beans

This gentle cooking method keeps the chicken breast moist and flavorful. Roasted sweet potato and green beans add vibrant color and essential nutrients.

Ingredients:

- 2 boneless, skinless chicken breasts

- 4 cups low-sodium chicken broth

- 1 bay leaf

- 4 sprigs fresh thyme

- 1 large sweet potato, peeled and cubed

- 1 cup trimmed green beans

- Salt and pepper to taste

Instructions:

1. Preheat oven to 400°F (200°C). Lightly grease a baking sheet.

2. In a large pot, bring chicken broth, bay leaf, and thyme sprigs to a simmer.

3. Add chicken breasts and poach for 15-20 minutes, or until cooked through.

4. While the chicken is poaching, toss sweet potato cubes with a drizzle of olive oil and season with salt and pepper. Spread them on the prepared baking sheet and roast for 20-25 minutes, or until tender-crisp.

5. Add green beans to the simmering broth with the chicken for the last 5 minutes of cooking.

6. Remove chicken from the broth and let cool slightly before shredding.

7. Serve shredded chicken with roasted sweet potato, green beans, and a bit of the poaching broth (optional).

Nutritional Information (per serving):

- Calories: 400

- Protein: 35g

- Fat: 5g

- Carbs: 50g

4. Shrimp Scampi with Zucchini Noodles

This light and flavorful dish features shrimp simmered in a garlicky lemon sauce, served over zucchini noodles for a low-fiber alternative to traditional pasta.

Ingredients:

- 1 pound shrimp, peeled and deveined

- 1 tablespoon olive oil

- 3 cloves garlic, minced

- 1/2 cup dry white wine

- 1 cup low-sodium chicken broth

- 1 tablespoon lemon juice

- 1/4 teaspoon dried parsley

- Salt and pepper to taste

- 2 large zucchinis

Instructions:

1. Heat olive oil in a large skillet over medium heat. Add garlic and cook for 30 seconds, until fragrant.

2. Add shrimp and cook for 2-3 minutes per side, or until pink and opaque. Remove shrimp from the pan and set aside.

3. Pour white wine into the pan and scrape up any browned bits. Let the wine simmer for 1 minute.

4. Add chicken broth, lemon juice, and parsley. Bring to a simmer and cook for 5 minutes.

5. Season with salt and pepper to taste.

6. Using a spiralizer or julienne peeler, create zucchini noodles from the zucchinis.

7. Add zucchini noodles to the pan with the sauce and cook for 2-3 minutes, or until heated through.

8. Return shrimp to the pan and toss to coat in the sauce.

9. Serve shrimp scampi over zucchini noodles.

Nutritional Information (per serving):

- Calories: 350

- Protein: 30g

- Fat: 10g

- Carbs: 15g

5. Baked Salmon Burgers with Avocado Crema

These salmon burgers are a delicious and healthy alternative to beef burgers. Topped with a creamy avocado crema, they're packed with flavor and protein.

Ingredients:

- 1 pound salmon fillet, skin removed and chopped

- 1/4 cup panko breadcrumbs

- 1/4 cup chopped red onion

- 1 tablespoon chopped fresh dill

- 1 egg, beaten

- Salt and pepper to taste

- Hamburger buns (preferably whole-wheat)

- Avocado Crema (recipe below)

For the Avocado Crema:

- 1/2 avocado, mashed

- 1/4 cup plain Greek yogurt

- 1 tablespoon lemon juice

- 1/4 cup chopped fresh cilantro

- Salt and pepper to taste

Instructions:

1. Preheat oven to 400°F (200°C). Line a baking sheet with parchment paper.

2. In a large bowl, combine chopped salmon, panko breadcrumbs, red onion, dill, egg, salt, and pepper. Mix well to combine.

3. Form the salmon mixture into burger patties.

4. Place salmon burgers on the prepared baking sheet and bake for 12-15 minutes, or until cooked through.

5. While the salmon burgers are baking, prepare the avocado crema. In a bowl, mash together avocado, Greek yogurt, lemon juice, cilantro, salt, and pepper.

6. Toast hamburger buns, if desired.

7. Serve salmon burgers on buns topped with avocado crema.

Nutritional Information (per serving with whole-wheat bun):

- Calories: 500
- Protein: 40g
- Fat: 20g
- Carbs: 35g

6. Chicken Stir-Fry with Snow Peas and Carrots

This quick and easy stir-fry is packed with protein and vegetables. Snow peas and carrots offer a low-fiber alternative to traditional stir-fry vegetables.

Ingredients:

- 1 pound boneless, skinless chicken breasts, cut into strips
- 1 tablespoon cornstarch
- 2 tablespoons soy sauce (low-sodium)
- 1 tablespoon rice vinegar

- 1 tablespoon sesame oil

- 1 cup snow peas

- 2 carrots, julienned

- 1 tablespoon olive oil

- Cooked brown rice (optional)

Instructions:

1. In a bowl, toss chicken strips with cornstarch, soy sauce, rice vinegar, and sesame oil.

2. Heat olive oil in a large skillet or wok over medium-high heat. Add chicken and cook for 5-7 minutes, or until browned and cooked through.

3. Add snow peas and carrots to the pan and cook for an additional 2-3 minutes or until tender-crisp.

4. Serve chicken stir-fry over cooked brown rice (optional).

Nutritional Information (per serving without rice):

- Calories: 300

- Protein: 35g

- Fat: 10g

- Carbs: 15g

7. One-Pan Lemon Garlic Shrimp with Asparagus

This sheet-pan dinner is a breeze to clean up! Shrimp and asparagus are roasted together with a simple lemon garlic sauce, making for a flavorful and protein-rich meal.

Ingredients:

- 1 pound shrimp, peeled and deveined

- 1 bunch asparagus, trimmed

- 1 tablespoon olive oil

- 1 tablespoon lemon juice

- 1 teaspoon minced garlic

- 1/4 teaspoon dried oregano

- Salt and pepper to taste

Instructions:

1. Preheat oven to 400°F (200°C). Line a baking sheet with parchment paper.

2. In a bowl, toss shrimp, asparagus, olive oil, lemon juice, garlic, oregano, salt, and pepper.

3. Spread the shrimp and asparagus mixture on the prepared baking sheet.

4. Roast for 10-12 minutes, or until shrimp are pink and opaque and asparagus is tender-crisp.

Nutritional Information (per serving):

- Calories: 300

- Protein: 30g

- Fat: 10g

- Carbs: 10g

8. Turkey Chili with Corn and Bell Peppers

This hearty chili is packed with lean protein and vegetables. Corn and bell peppers add a touch of sweetness and vibrant color. Serve with a side salad for a complete meal.

Ingredients:

- 1 tablespoon olive oil

- 1 pound ground turkey

- 1 onion, chopped

- 2 cloves garlic, minced

- 1 (28-ounce) can crushed tomatoes, undrained

- 1 (15-ounce) can kidney beans, drained and rinsed

- 1 (15-ounce) can black beans, drained and rinsed

- 1 (15-ounce) can corn, drained

- 1 red bell pepper, chopped

- 1 green bell pepper, chopped

- 1 tablespoon chili powder

- 1 teaspoon ground cumin

- 1/2 teaspoon dried oregano

- Salt and pepper to taste

Instructions:

1. Heat olive oil in a large pot or Dutch oven over medium heat. Add ground turkey and cook until browned, breaking it up with a spoon as it cooks.

2. Add onion and garlic and cook for an additional minute, until softened.

3. Stir in crushed tomatoes, kidney beans, black beans, corn, bell peppers, chili powder, cumin, oregano, salt, and pepper.

4. Bring to a boil, then reduce heat and simmer for 30 minutes, or until thickened.

5. Serve chili hot with a side salad (optional).

Nutritional Information (per serving):

- Calories: 400

- Protein: 30g

- Fat: 15g

- Carbs: 40g

9. Salmon with Mango Salsa and Coconut Rice

This tropical-inspired dish features flavorful grilled salmon topped with a refreshing mango salsa. Coconut rice adds a touch of sweetness and complements the salmon perfectly.

Ingredients:

- **For the Salmon:**

    o 2 salmon fillets (around 6 oz each)

    o 1 tablespoon olive oil

    o Salt and pepper to taste

- **For the Mango Salsa:**

    o 1 ripe mango, diced

    o 1/4 cup red onion, diced

    o 1/4 cup chopped fresh cilantro

- o   1 tablespoon lime juice

- o   Salt and pepper to taste

- **For the Coconut Rice:**

  - o   1 cup basmati rice

  - o   1 (13.5-ounce) can coconut milk

  - o   1/2 cup water

  - o   1/4 teaspoon salt

Instructions:

1. Preheat grill to medium-high heat.

2. For the mango salsa, combine diced mango, red onion, cilantro, lime juice, salt, and pepper in a bowl. Set aside.

3. For the coconut rice, rinse basmati rice in a fine-mesh strainer. In a saucepan, combine rice, coconut milk, water, and salt. Bring to a boil, then reduce heat, cover, and simmer for 15-20 minutes, or until rice is cooked and fluffy. Fluff the rice with a fork before serving.

4. Brush salmon fillets with olive oil and season with salt and pepper.

5. Grill salmon for 4-5 minutes per side, or until cooked through and flakes easily with a fork.

6. Serve grilled salmon over coconut rice and top with mango salsa.

Nutritional Information (per serving):

- Calories: 500

- Protein: 35g

- Fat: 20g

- Carbs: 40g

10. Grilled Chicken Caprese Salad

This deconstructed salad combines grilled chicken, fresh mozzarella, tomatoes, and a balsamic glaze for a light and flavorful meal.

Ingredients:

- 2 boneless, skinless chicken breasts

- 1 tablespoon olive oil

- Salt and pepper to taste

- 1 ball fresh mozzarella, sliced

- 2 large tomatoes, sliced

- 1/4 cup chopped fresh basil

- Balsamic glaze (store-bought or homemade)

Instructions:

1. Preheat grill to medium-high heat.

2. Brush chicken breasts with olive oil and season with salt and pepper.

3. Grill chicken for 5-7 minutes per side, or until cooked through.

4. While the chicken is cooking, arrange sliced mozzarella and tomatoes on a plate.

5. Once cooked, slice the chicken breast and arrange it on top of the mozzarella and tomatoes.

6. Sprinkle with chopped fresh basil.

7. Drizzle with balsamic glaze to taste.

Nutritional Information (per serving):

- Calories: 400

- Protein: 40g

- Fat: 15g

- Carbs: 20g

These EPI-friendly dinner recipes offer a variety of flavorful and satisfying options to end your day on a healthy note. Enjoy!

Chapter Seven

EPI-Friendly Snack Delights:

These snack recipes provide a delicious and satisfying way to curb your hunger between meals while managing your EPI. They focus on healthy fats, complex carbohydrates, and lean protein sources, keeping you energized and comfortable.

1. Apple Slices with Almond Butter

This classic snack combines the sweetness of apples with the protein and healthy fats of almond butter. It's a simple yet satisfying option.

Ingredients:

- 1 apple, sliced

- 2 tablespoons almond butter

Instructions:

1. Wash and slice the apple.

2. Spread almond butter on apple slices or enjoy them for dipping.

Nutritional Information (per serving):

- Calories: 200

- Protein: 5g

- Fat: 10g

- Carbs: 25g

2. Cottage Cheese with Berries and Chia Seeds

This protein-packed snack is full of flavor and texture. Cottage cheese provides protein and calcium, while berries add a touch of sweetness and antioxidants. Chia seeds offer a boost of fiber and healthy fats.

Ingredients:

- 1/2 cup low-fat cottage cheese

- 1/4 cup mixed berries (blueberries, raspberries, strawberries)

- 1 tablespoon chia seeds

Instructions:

1. In a bowl, combine cottage cheese, berries, and chia seeds.

2. Stir gently to combine and enjoy.

Nutritional Information (per serving):

- Calories: 150

- Protein: 15g

- Fat: 3g

- Carbs: 10g

3. Turkey Roll-Ups with Hummus and Vegetables

These protein-rich roll-ups are a great way to satisfy your hunger cravings. Lean turkey breast is paired with creamy hummus and crunchy vegetables for a delicious and balanced snack.

Ingredients:

- 4 slices deli turkey breast

- 1/4 cup hummus

- Baby carrots, sliced cucumber, or bell pepper strips
  (optional)

Instructions:

1. Spread hummus evenly over each slice of turkey
   breast.

2. Add your desired vegetables (baby carrots, sliced
   cucumber, or bell pepper strips) to the center of the
   turkey slice.

3. Roll up the turkey breast tightly and enjoy.

Nutritional Information (per serving with vegetables):

- Calories: 250

- Protein: 20g

- Calories: 250

- Protein: 20g

- Fat: 5g

- Carbs: 15g

4. Greek Yogurt Parfait with Granola and Berries

This layered parfait is a delicious and nutritious way to satisfy your sweet tooth. Greek yogurt provides protein and calcium, while granola adds complex carbohydrates and healthy fats. Berries offer a burst of sweetness and antioxidants.

Ingredients:

- 1/2 cup plain Greek yogurt

- 1/4 cup granola (choose a low-fiber option)

- 1/4 cup mixed berries (blueberries, raspberries, strawberries)

Instructions:

1. In a small glass or container, layer Greek yogurt, granola, and berries.

2. Repeat layers for a visually appealing parfait.

3. Enjoy chilled.

Nutritional Information (per serving):

- Calories: 250

- Protein: 15g

- Fat: 5g

- Carbs: 30g

5. Hard-Boiled Eggs with Edamame

This protein-packed snack is simple yet satisfying. Hard-boiled eggs are a great source of lean protein, while edamame adds a touch of plant-based protein, healthy fats, and fiber (in moderation for EPI).

Ingredients:

- 2 hard-boiled eggs

- 1/2 cup shelled edamame (optional, steamed or frozen)

Instructions:

1. Peel the hard-boiled eggs.

2. Enjoy the eggs on their own or pair them with steamed or frozen edamame for a more substantial snack.

Nutritional Information (per serving without edamame):

- Calories: 150

- Protein: 12g

- Fat: 10g

- Carbs: 1g

Nutritional Information (per serving with edamame):

- Calories: 200

- Protein: 18g

- Fat: 5g

- Carbs: 10g (be mindful of portion size for edamame)

6. Cucumber Slices with Smoked Salmon and Cream Cheese

This elegant and flavorful snack is perfect for a light bite. Cucumber slices provide a refreshing base, while smoked salmon offers a rich protein source. A touch of cream cheese adds creaminess without being heavy.

Ingredients:

- 1 cucumber, sliced

- 2 ounces smoked salmon

- 1 tablespoon light cream cheese

Instructions:

1. Spread a thin layer of cream cheese on each cucumber slice.

2. Top with a piece of smoked salmon.

3. Enjoy!

Nutritional Information (per serving):

- Calories: 150

- Protein: 10g

- Fat: 5g

- Carbs: 5g

7. Roasted Chickpeas with Spices

These crunchy and flavorful roasted chickpeas are a healthy alternative to chips. They're packed with protein and fiber (in moderation for EPI) and can be seasoned with various spices to suit your taste.

Ingredients:

- 1 can (15 oz) chickpeas, drained and rinsed

- 1 tablespoon olive oil

- 1/2 teaspoon dried cumin

- 1/4 teaspoon smoked paprika

- Salt and pepper to taste

Instructions:

1. Preheat oven to 400°F (200°C). Line a baking sheet with parchment paper.

2. Pat the chickpeas dry with a paper towel.

3. In a bowl, toss chickpeas with olive oil, cumin, paprika, salt, and pepper.

4. Spread the chickpeas on the prepared baking sheet in a single layer.

5. Roast for 20-25 minutes, or until golden brown and crispy.

6. Let cool slightly before enjoying.

Nutritional Information (per serving):

- Calories: 200

- Protein: 8g

- Fat: 5g

- Carbs: 20g (be mindful of portion size)

8. Rice Cakes with Avocado and Sliced Tomato

This simple snack combines healthy fats from avocado with complex carbohydrates from rice cakes and a touch of vitamin C from tomato.

Ingredients:

- 2 small rice cakes

- 1/4 avocado, sliced

- 1 slice tomato

Instructions:

1. Spread sliced avocado on each rice cake.

2. Top with a slice of tomato.

3. Enjoy!

Nutritional Information (per serving):

- Calories: 150

- Protein: 1g

- Fat: 10g

- Carbs: 20g

9. Bell Pepper Strips with Guacamole

This vibrant snack offers a satisfying combination of crunch and creaminess. Bell pepper strips provide a source of vitamin C, while guacamole adds healthy fats and a touch of protein.

Ingredients:

- 1 red or yellow bell pepper, sliced into strips

- 1/4 cup guacamole (prepared or make your own with mashed avocado, lime juice, and a pinch of salt)

Instructions:

1. Slice the bell pepper into strips.

2. Serve the bell pepper strips with a side of guacamole for dipping.

Nutritional Information (per serving):

- Calories: 150

- Protein: 2g

- Fat: 10g

- Carbs: 15g

10. String Cheese with Grapes

This classic snack pairing offers a balance of protein and carbohydrates. String cheese provides a convenient source of protein, while grapes add a touch of sweetness and fiber (in moderation for EPI).

Ingredients:

- 1 string cheese stick

- 1/4 cup grapes

Instructions:

1. Enjoy the string cheese and grapes together.

Nutritional Information (per serving):

- Calories: 150

- Protein: 8g

- Fat: 5g

- Carbs: 20g (be mindful of portion size for grapes)

These EPI-friendly snack recipes provide a variety of delicious and satisfying options to keep you energized and comfortable throughout the day. Remember to choose portion sizes that suit your individual needs and preferences. Enjoy!

Chapter Eight

EPI-Friendly Delights: Sweet Endings

These dessert recipes offer a satisfying way to finish your meal while keeping your EPI in mind. They focus on low-fiber fruits, lean protein sources, and minimal added sugars for a guilt-free treat.

1. Baked Pears with Ricotta and Honey

This elegant dessert features juicy baked pears topped with a creamy ricotta cheese mixture and a drizzle of honey.

Ingredients:

- 2 ripe pears

- 1/4 cup ricotta cheese

- 1 tablespoon honey

- 1/4 teaspoon ground cinnamon

- Fresh mint leaves for garnish (optional)

Instructions:

1. Preheat oven to 375°F (190°C).

2. Core the pears, leaving the bottoms intact.

3. In a small bowl, combine ricotta cheese, honey, and cinnamon.

4. Fill the pear cavities with the ricotta mixture.

5. Place the pears in a baking dish and bake for 20-25 minutes, or until the pears are tender and the filling is slightly golden.

6. Let cool slightly before serving. Garnish with fresh mint leaves (optional).

Nutritional Information (per serving):

- Calories: 200

- Protein: 5g

- Fat: 5g

- Carbs: 30g

2. Protein Smoothie with Berries and Spinach

This refreshing smoothie is a delicious and nutritious way to satisfy your sweet tooth. It packs a protein punch with Greek yogurt and offers a touch of fiber from spinach (in moderation for EPI).

Ingredients:

- 1 cup plain Greek yogurt

- 1/2 cup frozen berries (blueberries, raspberries, strawberries)

- 1/4 cup unsweetened almond milk

- 1/4 cup baby spinach (optional)

- 1/2 teaspoon vanilla extract

- Stevia or monk fruit sweetener to taste (optional)

Instructions:

1. Combine all ingredients in a blender and blend until smooth and creamy.

2. Taste and add stevia or monk fruit sweetener if desired.

3. Pour into a glass and enjoy!

Nutritional Information (per serving):

- Calories: 200

- Protein: 20g

- Fat: 5g

- Carbs: 20g (be mindful of portion size for spinach)

3. Poached Pears with Vanilla Sauce

This light and elegant dessert features poached pears in a flavorful vanilla sauce.

Ingredients:

- **For the Pears:**

    o 2 ripe pears

    o 2 cups water

    o 1/4 cup sugar

- o   1/2 vanilla bean, split lengthwise

- **For the Vanilla Sauce:**

  - o   1 cup low-fat milk

  - o   1 egg yolk

  - o   1 tablespoon cornstarch

  - o   1/4 teaspoon vanilla extract

Instructions:

1. In a saucepan, combine water, sugar, and vanilla bean. Bring to a simmer.

2. Peel the pears, leaving the stems intact. Add them to the simmering liquid.

3. Poach the pears for 15-20 minutes, or until tender.

4. While the pears are poaching, prepare the vanilla sauce. In a small saucepan, whisk together milk, egg yolk, and cornstarch.

5. Cook over medium heat, whisking constantly, until the mixture thickens and begins to simmer.

6. Remove from heat and stir in vanilla extract.

7. Let the pears cool slightly in the poaching liquid.

8. Serve pears with the vanilla sauce spooned over them.

Nutritional Information (per serving):

- Calories: 250

- Protein: 2g

- Fat: 5g

- Carbs: 40g

4. Angel Food Cake with Berries and Whipped Cream

This classic dessert is light and airy, making it a perfect EPI-friendly treat. Top it with fresh berries and a dollop of whipped cream for extra flavor.

Ingredients:

- 1 store-bought angel food cake (choose a low-fat option if available)

- 1 cup fresh berries (blueberries, raspberries, strawberries)

- 1 cup low-fat whipped cream

Instructions:

1. Slice the angel food cake into serving pieces.

2. Arrange the cake slices on plates.

3. Top with fresh berries and a dollop of whipped cream.

Nutritional Information (per serving):

- Calories: 300

- Protein: 3g

- Fat: 5g

- Carbs: 45g

5. Baked Apples with a Sprinkle of Cinnamon

This classic dessert is a perfect example of how delicious and satisfying EPI-friendly meals can be. Baked apples are naturally low in fiber and fat, making them a great choice for people managing Exocrine Pancreatic Insufficiency. The addition of cinnamon provides a touch of warmth and sweetness without added sugars.

Ingredients:

- 2 apples (choose a variety with a firm flesh, such as Granny Smith, Honeycrisp, or Gala)

- 1/4 teaspoon ground cinnamon

Instructions:

1. Preheat oven to 375°F (190°C).

2. Wash the apples and dry them thoroughly.

3. Using a sharp knife, core the apples from the top, leaving the bottom intact. You can use a spoon or melon baller to carefully scoop out the core, creating a hollow center.

4. (Optional) For added stability, you can slice a thin layer off the bottom of each apple so they sit flat in the baking dish.

5. Sprinkle the inside of each apple cavity with ground cinnamon.

6. Place the apples in a baking dish. You can add a splash of water (about 1/4 cup) to the bottom of the dish to prevent them from drying out.

7. Bake for 20-25 minutes, or until the apples are tender when pierced with a fork. The skins should be slightly wrinkled but not burst.

8. Let the apples cool slightly before serving. You can enjoy them warm or at room temperature.

Tips:

- For a touch of extra sweetness, drizzle the baked apples with a teaspoon of honey or maple syrup before serving. Be mindful of portion sizes for added sugars.

- Get creative with toppings! You can add a dollop of low-fat whipped cream, a sprinkle of chopped nuts, or a handful of fresh berries for a more decadent dessert.

- Leftover baked apples can be stored in an airtight container in the refrigerator for up to 3 days. Reheat them gently in the microwave before serving.

Nutritional Information (per serving):

- Calories: 100

- Protein: 0g

- Fat: 0g

- Carbs: 25g (mostly natural sugars from the apples)

6. Greek Yogurt Parfait with Mango and Chia Seeds

This layered parfait offers a delicious and nutritious combination of protein and healthy fats.

Ingredients:

- 1/2 cup plain Greek yogurt

- 1/4 cup chopped mango

- 1 tablespoon chia seeds

Instructions:

1. In a small glass or container, layer Greek yogurt, chopped mango, and chia seeds.

2. Repeat layers for a visually appealing parfait.

3. Enjoy chilled.

Nutritional Information (per serving):

- Calories: 200

- Protein: 15g

- Fat: 5g

- Carbs: 20g

7. Chocolate Chia Seed Pudding

This creamy pudding is a healthy and satisfying way to enjoy a chocolatey treat. Chia seeds provide fiber (in moderation for EPI) and healthy fats, while cocoa powder adds a touch of chocolate flavor.

Ingredients:

- 1 cup unsweetened almond milk

- 1/4 cup chia seeds

- 1 tablespoon unsweetened cocoa powder

- 1/2 teaspoon vanilla extract

- Stevia or monk fruit sweetener to taste (optional)

Instructions:

1. In a bowl or jar, combine almond milk, chia seeds, cocoa powder, and vanilla extract.

2. Stir well and refrigerate for at least 2 hours, or overnight, to allow the chia seeds to thicken.

3. Before serving, taste and add stevia or monk fruit sweetener if desired.

Nutritional Information (per serving):

- Calories: 200

- Protein: 4g

- Fat: 8g

- Carbs: 15g (be mindful of portion size for chia seeds)

8. Frozen Banana Bites with Nut Butter

These healthy and delicious frozen treats are perfect for satisfying a sweet tooth. Bananas provide natural sweetness and potassium, while nut butter adds protein and healthy fats.

Ingredients:

- 2 ripe bananas, peeled and sliced

- 2 tablespoons nut butter (almond butter, peanut butter, or cashew butter)

Instructions:

1. Line a baking sheet with parchment paper.

2. Arrange the banana slices on the prepared baking sheet in a single layer.

3. Freeze for at least 2 hours, or until frozen solid.

4. Drizzle or dip the frozen banana slices in nut butter before enjoying.

Nutritional Information (per serving):

- Calories: 200

- Protein: 3g

- Fat: 8g

- Carbs: 25g

9. Baked Apples with Cranberries and Walnuts

This warm and comforting dessert features baked apples filled with a mixture of tart cranberries and crunchy walnuts.

Ingredients:

- 2 apples

- 1/4 cup dried cranberries

- 1/4 cup chopped walnuts

- 1 tablespoon honey

- 1/4 teaspoon ground cinnamon

- 1/4 teaspoon ground ginger (optional)

- Pinch of nutmeg (optional)

Instructions:

1. Preheat oven to 375°F (190°C).

2. Core the apples, leaving the bottoms intact.

3. In a small bowl, combine dried cranberries, chopped walnuts, honey, cinnamon, ginger (if using), and nutmeg (if using).

4. Stuff the apple cavities with the cranberry-walnut mixture.

5. Place the apples in a baking dish and bake for 25-30 minutes, or until the apples are tender and the filling is bubbly.

6. Let cool slightly before serving.

Nutritional Information (per serving):

- Calories: 300

- Protein: 2g

- Fat: 8g

- Carbs: 40g

10. Melon Ball Skewers with Mint

This refreshing and light dessert is perfect for a warm day. Honeydew melon and cantaloupe offer natural sweetness and hydration, while mint leaves add a touch of freshness.

Ingredients:

- 1 cup honeydew melon, cut into balls
- 1 cup cantaloupe, cut into balls
- Fresh mint leaves for garnish

Instructions:

1. Using a melon baller, scoop out balls from the honeydew melon and cantaloupe.
2. Thread the melon balls onto skewers, alternating between honeydew and cantaloupe.
3. Garnish with fresh mint leaves.

Nutritional Information (per serving):

- Calories: 50

- Protein: 0g

- Fat: 0g

- Carbs: 15g

These EPI-friendly dessert recipes provide a variety of delicious and satisfying options to end your meal on a sweet note. Remember to choose portion sizes that suit your individual needs and preferences. Enjoy!

Chapter Nine

Lifestyle Strategies for Managing EPI

Living with EPI requires a proactive approach to managing your condition. This chapter explores various lifestyle strategies that can significantly improve your overall health and well-being.

Importance of Exercise for Overall Health and EPI Management

Regular exercise offers a multitude of benefits for people with EPI, beyond just maintaining a healthy weight. Here's how:

- **Improved Digestion:** Physical activity stimulates the digestive system, promoting smoother food movement and potentially reducing cramping and bloating.

- **Enhanced Nutrient Absorption:** Exercise can improve the body's ability to absorb essential nutrients from food, which is crucial for overall health, especially when dealing with digestive limitations.

- **Increased Energy Levels:** Regular exercise combats fatigue, a common symptom of EPI. Physical activity boosts energy production and overall well-being.

- **Stress Reduction:** Exercise is a natural stress reliever. By managing stress levels, you can potentially minimize digestive flare-ups associated with anxiety.

- **Muscle Strengthening:** Maintaining muscle mass is important for digestion and overall health. Exercise helps build and maintain muscle strength.

Finding the Right Exercise:

- **Focus on Low-Impact Activities:** Choose exercises that are gentle on your digestive system, such as walking, swimming, yoga, or cycling.

- **Listen to Your Body:** Start slowly and gradually increase the intensity and duration of your workouts as tolerated.

- **Consult Your Doctor:** Discuss your exercise plans with your doctor to ensure they are safe and appropriate for your specific condition.

Stress Management Techniques for EPI Patients

Stress can significantly worsen EPI symptoms. Here are some effective stress-management techniques:

- **Relaxation Techniques:** Practice deep breathing exercises, meditation, or progressive muscle relaxation to calm your mind and body.

- **Mindfulness Techniques:** Mindfulness practices like yoga or guided meditation can help you focus on the present moment and reduce stress-related anxiety.

- **Cognitive Behavioral Therapy (CBT):** CBT can help identify and change negative thought patterns that contribute to stress.

- **Getting Enough Sleep:** Adequate sleep promotes a healthy stress response. Aim for 7-8 hours of quality sleep each night.

- **Building a Support System:** Surround yourself with supportive friends, family, and healthcare professionals who can offer encouragement and understanding.

Traveling with EPI

Traveling with EPI requires additional planning, but it is still possible. Here are some tips:

- **Plan Ahead:** Research your destination and identify restaurants with suitable menu options or grocery stores where you can stock up on safe foods.

- **Pack Your Enzyme Supplements:** Ensure you have enough enzyme replacements to last throughout your trip, with some extras in case of delays.

- **Maintain a Regular Routine:** As much as possible, stick to your regular eating and medication schedule to minimize digestive disruptions.

- **Stay Hydrated:** Drink plenty of bottled water throughout your travels to avoid dehydration, which can worsen symptoms.

- **Be Flexible:** Unexpected situations may arise. Be prepared to adapt your plans and remain calm if digestive issues occur.

Building a Support Network

Living with EPI can be challenging. Building a strong support network can significantly improve your overall well-being. Here's how:

- **Connect with EPI Support Groups:** Joining online or in-person support groups allows you to connect with others who understand your experiences.

- **Talk to Your Doctor:** Open communication with your doctor is key. Discuss your concerns and work together to develop a management plan that suits your needs.

- **Lean on Loved Ones:** Share your challenges with supportive family and friends. Having a listening ear and a shoulder to lean on can make a big difference.

By incorporating these lifestyle strategies into your daily routine, you can effectively manage your EPI and experience a significant improvement in your overall health and quality of life. Remember, you are not alone. With the right approach and support system, you can thrive with EPI.

Chapter Ten

Appendix

This appendix provides additional resources to support you on your journey with EPI.

Glossary of Terms

- **Entrées:** Main courses of a meal.

- **Exocrine Pancreas:** The part of the pancreas that releases digestive enzymes.

- **Fiber:** A type of carbohydrate that aids digestion and promotes gut health. (**Note:** People with EPI may need to limit fiber intake in moderation).

- **Flare-up:** A sudden worsening of symptoms.

- **Malabsorption:** The inability to absorb nutrients properly from food.

- **Pancreatitis:** Inflammation of the pancreas.

- **Steatorrhea:** Fatty stools, a common symptom of EPI.

- **Supplements:** Additional nutrients or enzymes taken by mouth.

Sample Grocery Shopping List (EPI-Friendly Options)

Protein Sources:

- Lean meats (chicken breast, fish, turkey)

- Eggs

- Tofu or tempeh (in moderation)

- Low-fat dairy products (Greek yogurt, cottage cheese)

Fruits and Vegetables:

- Canned or cooked vegetables (easier to digest)

- Ripe fruits (bananas, berries, melons)

Grains and Starches:

- White rice

- Quinoa (in moderation)

- Potatoes (peeled and cooked)

- Gluten-free bread or pasta (if gluten intolerant)

Healthy Fats:

- Avocados

- Nuts and seeds (in moderation)

- Olive oil

Snacks:

- Hard-boiled eggs

- Rice cakes with nut butter and sliced banana

- Yogurt with berries and granola (choose low-fiber granola)

- Hummus with vegetable sticks

Remember: This is just a sample list. Be sure to discuss your specific dietary needs with your doctor or a registered dietitian.